THINGS
WE
EAT

By Opal Dockery

Things We Eat
By Opal Dockery
Copyright @ 2017 by Opal Dockery
First Printing 2017

Dixie Publishing Company
P.O. Box 364
Lamar, Missouri 64759

ISBN: 978-1-365-97704-6

Printed in the United States of America

I hope this very brief summary of "Thing We Eat" is of benefit to those who read it and encourage them to do further research.

THINGS WE EAT

When someone discovers that I am vegan they usually say,
"What do you eat?" I tell them, "Anything that is not animal
related." My son Jack, who is also vegan, answers the same
question, "Anything that does not have a mother." There are so
many **'THINGS WE EAT'** that it is impossible to consume all
of them in one week. I am quite certain I have forgotten some
of them; but I, at least, want to reveal the ones that I
do remember.

My Aunt Margaret used to say, "You need to eat something
you don't like everyday." She was referring to healthy foods.

I believe the "secret" to being healthy is to eat food that you
know is good for your health whether you like it or not. So
many will not eat food if they do not like the taste even though
the health benefits have been proven. Taste should not be an
issue when regarding health.

I eat so many foods I do not like, that sometimes I forget what I
do like. I am fine with this as long as I know they are healthy.
My son and I regard healthy food as medicine rather than just
food.

I thought it would be helpful to write a book explaining what
we eat and the reasons. I wish I had enough money to give this
book to each person who asks, "What do you eat?"

VEGAN
A vegan is a person who omits all animal products from the
diet and does not use any animal products such as leather
or wool. (144)

Basic List Of The 'THINGS WE EAT'

I am quite certain that I have forgotten some; but these are the ones I can remember at this time.

BEANS

BLACKSTRAP MOLASSES

BREAD

CHOCOLATE

COFFEE

CONDIMENTS
Bragg's Liquid Aminos
Soy Sauce
Tomato Ketchup
Veganaise
Yellow Mustard

FRUITS AND VEGETABLES
Fruits
Apples
Avocadoes
Bananas
Berries – (Blackberries, Blueberries, Raspberries)
Dates
Figs
Grapes
Lemons
Olives
Oranges
Prunes
Raisins
Tomatoes
Watermelon

Vegetables
Cruciferous Vegetables – (Broccoli, Brussels Sprouts, Cabbage, Cauliflower)
Bell Pepper
Carrots
Celery
Corn
Cucumbers
Dill Pickles
Garlic
Ginger
Horseradish
Kale
Mushrooms
Onions
Peas
Potatoes
Sauerkraut
Spinach

GRAINS
Couscous
Oatmeal
Popcorn
Quiona
Rice – (Brown, White)
Wheat Germ

JUICE
Cranberry Juice
Grape Juice
Orange Juice
Tomato Juice

LECHITHIN

MILK
Almond Milk
Soy Milk

NUTS
Almond Butter
Peanut Butter
Almonds
Brazil Nuts
Cashews
Hazelnuts
Macadamina Nuts
Peanuts
Pecans
Walnuts

OILS
Canola Oil
Coconut Oil
Olive Oil

SEEDS
Chia
Flaxseed
Heep Seed
Millet
Pumpkin Seeds
Sunflower Seeds

SALSA

SPAGHETTI

SPAGHETTI SAUCE

SPICES
Black Pepper
Cayenne Pepper
Cumin
Onion Powder
Par D' Arco
Salt
Turmeric

TEA
Chai Tea
Green Tea
Mint Medley Tea
Peppermint Tea
Smooth Move Tea

TOFU

VINEGAR
Apple Cider Vinegar
Bragg's Apple Cider Vinegar
Heinz Apple Cider Vinegar

WATER
Distilled And Purified

YEAST
Brewer's Yeast
Nutritional Yeast

The Following Is A Very Brief Summary Of The Research Which I Conducted Regarding The 'THINGS WE EAT'

BEANS, GRAINS, AND AMINO ACIDS

The Dietary Guidelines for Americans says we should eat more plant proteins. (1) Soybeans contain the most protein. They are the only bean that is a complete protein because they contain lysine which is an amino acid missing from other plant proteins. (3)

They are, also, composed of the most fat but are relatively low in calories. (8) Garbanzo beans have the lowest number of fat. All beans are great for dietary fiber. (5)

The daily requirement of protein for the average man, based on a 2,000 calorie diet, is 50 grams and 46 grams for an average woman. (4) One cup of soybeans provides 28.62 grams which is equal to 3 ounces of meat. White beans are the next highest with 17.42 grams in one cup. Others provide 15 to 17 grams in 1 cup while lima beans have only 10.32 grams. (3)

Although soybeans are the only beans with the complete protein, (6) when the wide variety of other beans are combined with foods such as grains like rice as well as corn and other vegetables, seeds, and nuts, a complete protein is evident and produces all the essental amino acids. Eating a combination of beans and particular foods, especially grains, is beneficial over eating these foods alone.

The major benefit of combining beans and grains comes from their amino acid contents. Both beans and grains, with the exception of soybeans, are examples of incomplete protein. They contain some, but not all, the essential amino acids. They also represent complementary proteins, which means that when you consume beans and grains together, their complementary amino acid contents provide your body with all the essential amino acids. For example, many grains are deficient in the essential amino acid lysine, a nutrient found in beans. Conversely, many beans contain only small amounts of methionine, an amino acid found in larger supply in grains.

Your body uses combinations of 20 types of amino acids to make protein, but not all these amino aids need to come from your diet. Only10 amino acids, termed essential amino acids, must come from the foods you eat while the remaining 10 nonessential amino acids can be synthesized within your cells. As a result, you should plan your diet to include all 10 essential amino acids to allow for proper protein synthesis. (7)

Protein plays a crucial role in almost all biological processes and amino acids are the building blocks of it. A large portion of our cells, muscles, and tissue is made up of amino acids, meaning they carry out many important bodily functions, such as giving cells their structure. They, also, play a key role in the transport and storage of nutrients. Amino acids have an influence on the function of organs, glands, tendons, and arteries. They are furthermore essential for healing wounds and repairing tissue especially in the muscles, bones, skin, and hair as well as for the removal of all kinds of waste deposits produced in connection with metabolism. (9)

Benefits Of Beans Are Many. Some Of Them Are:

Balances blood sugar: With a low glycemic index, beans contain a beautiful blend of complex carbohydrates and protein because they are digested slowly, which helps keep glucose stable and may curtail fatigue and irritability.
Convenient and versatile: Canned, frozen, or dry, beans are a breeze to purchase, prepare, and store. They, also, come in flour form. If canned, rinse off before cooking. This elimates 40 percent of sodium. (1)
Cuts cancer risks: Scientists recommend 3 cups per week to promote health and reduce the risk of chronic diseases like cancer due to their abundance of fiber and antioxidants. (2)

Gluten free: (5)

High degree of antioxidant protection: Red kidney beans rate higher than blueberries in this area. (1)

Lowers blood pressure: All beans and peas can help lower blood pressure due to their high content of fiber, poassium, and magnesium. (11)

Low in fat: They contain only 2 to 3 percent fat, which reinforces the fact that they contain no cholesterol, (1) and can lower cholesterol levels. (2) They are a good fat. A large percentage of the total fat consists of unsaturated fats and provides Omega-3 fats that fight inflammation (5)

Nutrient rich: Aside from protein, complex carbs, and fiber, beans contain a powerhouse of numerous nutrients. (1) As an example, just a half cup of black beans provides almost half the recommended daily requirements of iron for women and men who are over 50. (7)

Prevents constipation: Regulates the function of the colon and prevents piles as well as other bowel problems.

Satisfies you: Beans are metabolized more slowly than other complex carbs, which may aid in weight loss by keeping you feeling full without being excessively high in calories.

Soluble fiber: Can lower cholesterol and triglyceride levels, help the heart, (1) and lower the risk of cardiovascular disease. (2)

Super packed with protein: Just one half cup of beans equals 7 grams of protein which is the same amount as one third of chicken, fish, and meat.

Wallet friendly: Beans are the least expensive source of protein, especially, when compared to meat. (1) They have been called "the poor man's meat", but now are called "the rich man's meat"due to the discovery of their health benefits. (10)

We eat beans almost everyday. Although we like every kind of bean, pintos are our favorite.

On New Year's Day, we eat black-eyed peas before anything else as a tradition to bring 'good luck'.

Dry beans, instead of canned, are more heathy. Anyone who can boil water can cook dry beans. Just pour them on a flat surface like a plate or counter, take out any bad ones or rocks, rinse them really good, put them in a pot of water, and then cook them. Keep adding water as they cook; so they will not burn. If you soak them overnight, they swell-up and cook much faster.

I have discovered that a crockpot is the best way to cook them. But it is important to still add water every so often. My mother used to put them in a deep, flat cooking pan filled with water and bake them.

We usually cook a variety of beans together and usually add vegetables to the pot. Sometimes we add so many vegetables that it seems like a vegetable soup more than a pot of beans. When we add black-eyed peas, their favor overcomes the whole pot. Lentils are great to add for flavoring and thickness. especially, if you want to make vegetable soup.

We cook a whole pot of beans and make each bowl taste differently by adding a wide variety of things such as: Bragg's Amino Acids, soy sauce, veganaise, different grains or spices, vinegar, olive oil. garlic, or ginger to a hot bowl of beans. Or we just eat a bowl without adding anything. Cold beans by themselves tastes good, too.

We dip a bowl of beans from the pot each time we want some rather than heating the whole pot. Heating the whole batch over and over is not really healthy.

BLACKSTRAP MOLASSES
Helps prevent diabetes. It is a friendly sweetner and stabilizes blood sugar.
Bone booster – Has calcium and magnesium for bones – 5 tablespoons equal 50% of the recommended daily allowance of calcium, 95% of iron, 38% of magnesium which is crucial to prevent osteoporosis and asthma along with others that can affect your blood and heart

Very good for the blood
Packed with potassium (49)

Although blackstrap molasses is sweet, I really do not like the taste; but Jack does. We take a tablespoon regularly. I usually have a tablespoon every other day.

BREAD
It is quite difficult for us to find bread we can eat. Even though the package might say "vegan", if it reads that it is "processed in a facility that processes milk and eggs", we will not eat it. (142)

I cannot eat much bread because it constipates me. It does not bother Jack this way. He likes it better than I do.

CHOCOLATE
Dark Chocolate
Very nutritious
Rich in fiber and many minerals
Powerful source of antioxidants
May improve blood flow
Lowers blood pressure
Raises HDL and protects LDL against oxidation
Improves insulin sensitivity
Beneficial in lowering the risk of cardiovascular disease
Provides protection of your skin against the sun by improving blood flow to the skin
Can improve brain function (91)

It is extremely difficulty to find chocolate that was not processed in a facility that processes milk and eggs, even though the package says "vegan", which we cannot eat. Any food associated with the death of animals is off limits for our personal consumption.

The only store we have found that has the chocolate we can eat, is in our hometown of Lamar, Missouri. This store has three different kinds that we can eat. They charge $2.50 a bar, and it is worth every bite. We can order it on the internet for $9.00 and some cents plus shipping; but we have not become that desperate yet.

At times, we have gone for years without being able to eat chocolate. Although it is an extremely nice treat, we choose to live without it until we go to Lamar.

Dark chocolate is the most healthy of all chocolates.

COFFEE

Does not cause risk of heart disease
May help you live longer and lower risk of strokes
Biggest source of antioxidants in the Western Diet
Can cause small increase in blood pressure
Contains essential nutrients
Beneficial in lowering the risk of Type 2 diabetes
May protect against against Alzheimer's Disease and dementia
Good in lowering the risk of Parkinson's – 60% lower risk of getting it
Decreases the risk of cancer such as liver and colorectal cancer
Can fight against depression and make you happier
Reduces the risk of suicide
Great for brain function - Can improve energy levels and make you smarter
Burns fat
Drastically improves physical performance (90)

Even though I love to drink coffee, I can live without it. Many years ago, I decided to give up coffee which resulted in having withdrawals for two weeks; but it cured my desire. I started back just because I like the taste as well as the soothing effect it gives me. But I can get up in the morning and do without coffee all day without any cravings for it.

When I am hungry and do not want to eat, it helps to drink some coffee to curb my appetite.

Jack and I like to drink it together in the mornings and talk. We call it, "Our quality time".

Instead of doughnuts and coffee, we give ourselves a treat every so often and drink it with popcorn or chips. Although chips are not good for a person, occasionally, we do eat them. When Jack was a kid, he used to laugh at me because I ate chips with coffee. Now he likes to do the same. Avocados tastes great while drinking coffee,too.

When I drink a couple cups of natural coffee made from such ingredients like Chicory, I have no desire to have the regular coffee.

I do not like decaffinated coffee at all. If I drink coffee, I want the caffine in it.

Years ago, I used to put milk and sugar in my coffee which was causing me to gain weight because I drank so much. So I decided to learn to drink it black or not at all. Now I have no desire to put anything in it. I could not use milk anyway because it is an animal product, and I do not like sugar. I could use almond or soy milk, but I prefer not to usethem either. Jack has always drank his coffee black.

CONDIMENTS
Bragg Liquid Aminos

Made of only soybeans that have not been genetically modified and water, Bragg Liquid Aminos is a natural alternative to conventional soy sauces without the additional table salt, monosodium glutamate, preservatives, or gluten that can be found in many of the soy sauces on the market.

As the name implies, Bragg Liquid Aminos is an excellent source of amino acids made from soybeans used to make the seasoning. It contains 16 of the 20 amino acids, which are the building blocks of protein. Nine of the 20 amino acids cannot be produced by the body and need to be consumed through diet. (10), (15)

Soy Sauce
Antioxidant
Good for the immune and inflammatory system
Helps with Type 2 diabetes and allergies
Contains many vitamins
Has digestive tract benefits (34)

We use soy sauce probably more than Bragg's Amino Acids, mainly because it is so much handier to purchase. It is in all the grocery stores while Bragg's is usually available only in health food stores. But we like both of them.

We alternate between Bragg's Amino Acid and soy sauce. Although we usually buy only one at a time, sometimes we buy both. When we have both on hand, one day we might use Bragg's and the next day soy. Even though both are healthy, Bragg's is better for your health because it does not have as much sodium as soy and contains a cloudy looking substance that is called The Mother which is said to be very healthy. Both are good to add to salads or a hot bowl of beans. There is no need for salt, spices, or any other flavorings. But if you use too much they overcome the whole taste of the food.

Tomato Ketchup
Contains lycopene, a carotenoid and phytonutrient found in red fruits and vegetables like tomatoes
Prevents DNA damage in the cells
Reduces risk of cancer, including breast and prostate cancer, as well as heart disease, and macular degeneration
Promotes male fertility
Good for skin care, bone health, and vision (23)

Not only is this good for sandwiches, we use it as a dip. It, also, tastes good mixed with mustard as a dip. Ketchup adds flavor to a hot bowl of beans.

Veganaise
Has the texture of mayonaise but is much healthier
Free from eggs, dairy, gluten, trans fats, preservatives, and artificial ingredients
Heart-healthy with no GMOs (146)

We really like veganaise. It is good to add to a bowl of hot beans or soup, a salad, on a sandwich, or as a dip. Veganaise mixed with mustard is a good dip.

Our favorite is the "Original Follow Your Heart" made from soybeans. Many other natural spreads are available that compare to mayonaise. Trader's Joes sells a brand that tastes a lot like regular mayonaise.

Yellow Mustard
Contributes to digestive health
Allows a steady heart beat
Causes muscles to contract
Provides phosphorus which is found in every cell in the body, magnesium to process energy, and calcium to build teeth and bones
Good for the kidneys and heart functions
Very high in sodium
Has protein, fiber, and many vitamins including
C and B-complex (22)

We eat a lot of mustard. Not only is it good on sandwiches, we add it to salads, and use it as a dip. It, also, tastes good to mix it with ketchup or veganaise as a dip.

FRUITS AND VEGETABLES
Fruits and vegetables are rich in vitamins and minerals. Their natural antioxidants will help keep your body working at its best; so consuming a diet that meets your daily requirements of fruits and vegetables is one of the best ways to give your body a strong defense against disease.

Fruits and vegetables are protective to health. They lower high blood pressure and are helpful at reducing the risk of coronary heart disease, stroke, and some cancers. Other health benefits are the fact that they are low in calories, serving as an aid to prevent obesity, which is a significant risk factor for Type 2 diabetes, cancer, and cardiovascular disease. They contain a huge amount of fiber which fills you up and keeps your digestive system happy. (26)

You cannot eat too many fruits and vegetables. When we only eat raw fruits and vegetables we are never hungry. The body was designed to eat, exculsively, raw and nothing cooked.

Most people want to eat fruit as a desert; but it is best to eat fruit about thirty minutes before you eat. This helps clear the passage way for the rest of the meal.

FRUITS
All fruits have no cholesterol. (28)

I do not like fruit which is quite unusual for a vegan. The smell of them is repulsive, and it are so nasty. But I do like some such as tomatoes, avocadoes, olives, dates, and watermelon.

Although I hate fruit, I do eat a variety of it almost everyday because it is so healthy. I think of them as medicine. They are even healthier than vegetables which I really do like the best.

Jack does not feel the same way as I do regarding fruit. He likes it.

Apples

Contains fiber

Composed of carbs and water

Helps promote colon health

Controls blood sugar level – May help prevent diabetes

Protects against against heart disease

Lowers risk of cancer

Has many vitamins and minerals

High in various antioxidant compounds that are responsible for many health benefits

Weight loss – Low in calories (67)

This is the fruit I hate most of all, but I eat it a lot and really feel that it is the number one fruit that is good for you. I cut an apple up and mix it with anything I can to mask the taste and smell such as mustard, ketchup, or veganaise as well as soy sauce, olive oil, or apple cider vinegar. When I mix all these ingredients together, it really masks the taste.

One has to clean the skin really good to try getting rid of the chemicals used in the growing and processing apples.

Avocados

People who eat avocados tend to be healthy. They have a higher nutrient intake and a lower risk of metabolic syndrome.

Contains potassium and monosaturared fatty acids

Heart-healthy

Loaded with fiber

Lowers cholesterol and triglycerides levels

May help prevent cancer, lose weight, and relieve sympthoms of arthritis

Delicious and easy to incorporate into your diet

Provides a complete protein

Contains all the necessary amino-acids (27), (36)

Avocados contain all the amino acids necessary for good health. This is one fruit that both of us really like. We like to eat avocados with coffee instead of doughnuts.

Jack makes the best guacamole I have ever tasted. He will make a big bowl. When he does this, that is the only food we eat all day and have some left for the next day.

When I decide to eat only fruit for the day, I am glad that I like avocados. Also, when I decide to not eat at night, I allow myself to eat fruit. This is great to know that I can eat avocados at this time because they are a fruit.

Bananas
Even though bananas are technically berries, they are normally considered in the fruit category.
Contains many carbohydrates
Healthy antioxidants
Digestive health
Provides many vitamins and minerals
High in fiber (137)

Years ago I read a book about bananas which presented proof that they are the only food needed to maintain good health. I wish I still had that book or knew the name of it; so I could possibly buy it.

It is much easier for me to eat bananas than apples, but I do like to mix different things with them such as mustard or peanut butter in order to mask the taste and smell.

BERRIES

Fresh berries are the most disease-fighting foods available. Berries have some of the highest antioxidant levels of any fresh fruits. Kale and spinach are the only vegetable with antioxidant values as high as fresh berries. (100)

Berries are another fruit that I mask the taste with such things as mustard, ketchup, or soy sauce. Sometimes I put them in a hot cup of beans or a hot cup of tomato juice. Jack likes them by themselves.

Blackberries

Blackberries are, also, known as brambleberries, bramble, dewberry, thimbleberry, and lawers.
Highest antioxidant levels of all fruits.
Healthy tightening of the tissue to make skin look younger
Helps keep your brain alert
Reduces intestinal inflammation due to the high
tannin content (92)
If the blackberry plant turns orange, destroy it. This is a serious fungal disease that cannot be cured. (93)

Blackberries are considered the most healthful of all the berries according to many sources. But other sources such as the Dr. Oz Show claim that blueberries are the healthiest.

Although we both like these, Jack likes them better than I do. I like blueberries more than he does. But I still add things to mask the taste with both of them such as mustard, ketchup, or veganaise.

Blueberries

Reduces damage after strenuous exercise
Maintains brain function and improves memory
High in fiber
Anti-diabetic effects
Fights urinary tract infections
Low in calories
Provides many nutrients
85% water
Highest antioxidant of the wide variety of fruits and vegetables as well as all other foods
Reduces DNA damage, which may help protect against aging
Fights against cancer
Protects cholesterol in the blood from becoming damaged
Lowers blood pressure
Prevents heart disease (102)

Various sources such as the Dr. Oz Show claim that
blueberries are the healthiest berry. But other sources say
blackberries are. We like both of them. I like blueberries
more than Jack does. He likes blackberries more than I do.
Although I like both of them, I still mask them with such
things as mustard, ketchup, or veganaise.

Raspberries
Antioxidant and inflammatory benefits
Fights obesity
Controls blood sugar
Provides anti-cancer properties (101)

Raspberries are Jack's favorite. He likes them more than I do.
It is quite difficult to clean them. This has to be done very
gently because they break-apart so easily. You do not even
have to chew them – just mash them up in your mouth.
Although I like them, I still mask them with such things as
mustard, ketchup, or veganaise.

Dates
Promotes digestive health
Relieves constipation
Boosts heart health
Anti-inflammatory
Reduces blood pressure and strokes
Boosts brain health
Beneficial to a healthy pregnancy and delivery
Good source of fiber, vitamin B6, and many other
health benefits (48)

Although I do not care for sweets, dates are really good and
provide a naturally sweet taste. We like them very much.

Figs

Lowers blood pressure
Helps with losing weight
Protects against postmenopausal
Prevention against breast cancer
Beneficial effects on cardiovascular system
Lowers insulin
Reduces the risk of macular degeneration (47)

Figs taste really good. They provide a naturally sweet taste.
We like them very much.

Grapes

Grapes are biologically seeds.
One and a half cup equals 90 calories
Polyphenols are micronutrients that prevents degenerative
diseases. Resvertrol is a polypbenol found in the skin
of grapes.
Contains many antioxidants and vitamins
Has healthy carbs
High in fiber
Promotes colon health
Fights against heart disease
Aids with weight loss – Has no fat
Beneficial for eye health
Good for blood sugar and diabetes (73)

Grapes are one fruit I could live without. I really have to
mask the taste with such things as mustard, ketshup, or
veganaise. Jack likes them, but will only eat a few when we
buy them; therefore I eat the rest in order for them not to go to
waste. It is really difficut to gag them down. When Jack was
a kid, his favorite was the green ones.

Lemons

Lemons are the only food in the world that is anionic. It is anonic with a negative charge. All others are cationic (the ion has a postive charge). This makes it extremely useful to health as it is the intraction between anions and cations that ultimately promotes all cell energy.

When sufficient oxygen is unavaiable, like climbing mountains, lemons aid in the oxygen issue.

Lemons are the alkaline power food, alkalining the body. They are sour and warm, promoting gastric fire and light.

Lemons contain vitamin C which neutralizes free radicals linked to aging and most types of disease.

The lemon peel is effective for brain disorders like Parkinson's disease.

Dissolves gallstones, calcium deposits, and kidney stones

Contains powerful antioxidant properties and anti-cancer compounds

Good for the liver

Clears your bowels

Treats scurvy

Helps vision and eye disorders

Strengthens blood vessels

Destroys worms (38)

Lemons are one fruit we eat consistently. We peel it, cut it up, and eat the whole lemon. We, also, add it to salads. They are good to eat with avocados.

The lemon peeling is really heallhy. If you grate it or cut it in really thin pieces, you can add it to such foods as salads, soups, or a hot bowl of beans.

It is necessary for the skin to be cleaned really good in a effort to rid it of any chemicals.

Olives

The olive is a fruit.
74% of the fat is contain oleic acid, which is a
monounsaturated fatty acid that is the main component of
olive oil.
Decreases inflammation
Reduces risk of heart disease
Fights cancer
Low carb content which is mostly fiber
Contains many vitamins and minerals
Good for bone health
Provides the high antioxidant quercetin
Benefits blood pressure (103)

I could eat olives everyday. They are so good. I like all
kinds. Jack likes them, but not as much as I do.

I like to make an olive and mustard sandwich. When we used
to travel a lot, I ate these types of sandwiches quite frequently.
While on the road, we would stop at a truck stop for some
food. A jar of green olives was the only food I could find that
was vegan. Jack had no trouble finding something to eat
because he had not become vegan yet.

When we travel now, we take enough vegan food with us. We
take a laundry basket full of food when we drive which we
call our Food Basket. We usually take our coffee pot and
popcorn maker, too.

But when we travel on the Greyhound Bus, we can only take
enough food, which we put in a bag, to last us until we meet
our final destination.

Oranges
Contains carbs and water
Does not cause spikes in blood sugar
High in fiber
Promotes digestive health
Provides many vitamins and minerals
Helps prevent hearth disease
Reduces blood pressure
Promotes a blood thinning effect
Prevents kidney stones and anemia (70)

I mask the taste of these with such things as mustard, ketchup, or veganise. Jack likes them a lot.

The orange peeling is really healthy. If you grate it or cut it in really thin pieces, you can add it to such foods as salads, soups, or a hot bowl of beans.

It is necessary for the skin to be cleaned really good in a effort to rid it of any chemicals.

Prunes
Protects against cardiovascular diseases and other chronic illnesses
Helps prevent diabetes and obesity
Lowers cholesterol
Improves bones and reduces risk of osteoporosis
Good source of vitamin K and beta-carotene (51)

We do not like the taste of prunes, but we eat them because they are good for us. They are great for bowel movements.

Raisins

Helps prevent degenerative nerve disease, Alzheimer's and viral/fungal infections

Good source of B-complex vitamins

Gluten free

Contains many minerals

Provides antioxidant enzymes

High in anthocyanins that have anti-allergies, anti-inflammatory, anti-microbial, and anti-cancer activities

Required daily levels of dietary fiber

Lowers weight and cholesterol

Aids in preventing breast and colon cancer as well as constipation

Resveratrol – reduces risk of stroke

Good for the prostate

Lowers heart rate and blood pressure as well as being beneficial in preventing heart disease (50)

I do not like raisins, but just like the other fruits, I eat them. Jack likes them better than I do. I like to put them in a hot cup of tomato juice. This really fills me up and makes my bowels move really good the next day.

Tomatoes

Reduces heart disease

Rich in vitamins and minerals

Can reduce damage from smoking including second hand smoke

Naturally enhance flavor.

Dense in phytonutrients – few vegetables compare with tomatoes in this regard

Antioxidant

Organic tomatoes are king.

Promotes digestion and prevents constipation

Reduces dangers of statin drugs, in that, eating tomatoes may help you avoiding taking them

Prevents kidney and gall bladder stones
Beneficial for healthy hair and skin health
Good for bone health
Strengthens immune system
Reduces blood clot risks
Increases fat burning capacity
Protects vision and degenerative eye disease
Prevents stroke
Restores biochemical balance in diabetes
Reduces cancer risk of prostate and breast (86)

I love fresh tomatoes and could eat them everyday without getting tired of them. Jack does not like them; but he likes tomato products such as pasta sauce, salsa, and tomato juice.

Even though they are classified as fruits, I consider them as vegetables. But when I decide to eat only fruit for the day, I take advantage of this scientific fact and include tomatoes.

Also, when I decide to not eat at night, I allow myself to eat fruit. This is great to know that I can eat tomatoes at this time because they are a fruit.

Watermelon
91% water and 7.5% calories
Carbs are from the simple sugars.
Contains a small amount of fiber
Provides many vitamins and minerals
Lowers blood pressure
Beneficial for insulin resistance
Reduces muscle soreness after exercise
Good source of the amino acid citruline mostly found in the white rind and the antioxidant lycopene (82)

Watermelon is a fruit that I like a lot even though it is messy. It really fills me up and makes me pee a lot. Jack does not like this fruit at all.

When we buy watermelon, I have to eat the whole thing myself. Sometimes I just eat it and nothing else until there is none left.

VEGETABLES
I like all vegetables except Okra. It feels like I have a mouthfull of snot not matter how it is prepared. Jack likes it deep fried.

There are so many ways we eat vegetables such as raw, steamed, and stir-fried. Also, we really like cabbage and mustard sandwiches.

Cruciferous Vegetables
Are great for your health. One reason is due to their high sulfur content. Some of them are broccoli, Brussels Sprouts, cabbage, and cauliflower. (80)

These are my favorite vegtables.

Broccoli
Although cauliflower is very good for your health, broccoli has more nutrient value than cauliflower. (77)
The only carbs are in its fiber and sugar.
Provides gut health
Protein is low but higher than most other vegetables
Contains many vitamins and minerals
Good for cancer preventation
Lowers cholesterol
Promotes eye health
Benficial for the thyroid
Is a blood thinner (78)

All cruciferous vegetables are my favorite, but broccoli ranks as number one. Jack does not care for broccoli. But he will eat it.

Brussels Sprouts
Promotes detox support
Antioxidant
Reduces the risk of ulcerative colitis
Helps regulate inflammatory/anti-inflammatory system
Provides help for inflammatory bowel disease and irritable
bowel syndrome
Good for cardiovascular health
Aids in digestion
Beneficial for Crohn's disease
Is insulin resistance and is beneficial for Type 2 diabetes
Aids with the problem of obesity
Promotes in the help for rheumatoid arthritis (143)

Brussels Sprouts are so filling. It is difficult to stop eating
them. They taste so good when cooked without adding any
flavoring, but olive oil and apple cider vinegar added to them
taste good, too. It is difficult to eat them raw because they
have such a hard texture. We both like them so much.

Cabbage
Although all green cabbage is good for you, red cabbage has
more nutritional benefits such as unique antioxidants and
anti-inflammatory properties
Good for cancer prevention
Helps with the digestive tract
Beneficial for cardiovascular issues (79)

We use cabbage instead of lettuce in our salad. If I eat more
than a handfull of lettuce, I get a stomach ache. We really like
cabbage and mustard sandwiches.

Cauliflower

Although cauliflower is very good for your health, broccoli has more nutrient.
Fights cancer
Boosts heart health
Anti-inflammatory
Rich in vitamins and minerals
Beneficial for digestion
Antioxidants (77)

Cauliflower has a crispy taste when eaten raw. It tastes good anyway you eat it. We like it raw, steamed, microwaved, or boiled.

Bell Peppers

92% water
Most of the carbohydrates are sugar.
Small amounts of protein and fat
Has fiber
Contains many vitamins and minerals
Antioxidants
Good for eye health
Prevents anemia (88)

We like all bell peppers, but the green ones are our favorite. In the past we have used them in soup, but really do not like them that way. A green bell pepper and veganaise sandwich is really good.

Carrots

Mainly composed of water and carbohydrates
Antioxidant – beta-carotene
Has cardiovascular benefits
Helps in cancer prevention
Good for eye health
Lowers blood pressure
Aids in weight loss

High in fiber
Provides many vitamins and minerals (83)

I do not care that much for carrots. Jack likes them better than
celery while I like celery better than carrots. They tastes
better to me when I cut them into chunks and boil them.

When we juice, carrots are the only food we use. Raw carrots
make me thristy; so I eat a lot of them when I want to drink a
large amount of water.

Celery
Excellent source of antioxidants
Improves liver, skin, eyes, and cognitve health
Has electrolytes that prevents dehydration
Lowers blood pressure and inflammation
Beneficial fo irritable bowel syndrome
Helps prevent ulcers
Boosts digestion
Reduces bloating
Fights infections
Beneficial for urinary tract infections
Helps prevent cancer
Aids in weight loss (84)

Celery is a great snack and is really filling. We like to put
peanut or almond butter on it. Sometimes I cook a stalk of
celery with a pot of beans. It adds a flavor all to itself.

I like celery better than carrots while Jack likes carrots better
than celery.

Corn
Antioxidant
High fiber
Slowly digested source of carbohydrates
Gluten-free

Linked to longevity and overall health (105)
Provides a small amount of protein and fat
Contains many vitamins and minerals
Good for eye health
Prevents diverticular disease (106)

We like corn on the cob. Instead of butter, we use canola oil.
Jack likes this best. I like it too, but I also use olive oil and
veganaise. Jack just uses canola oil.

We do not like frozen corn. When we buy canned vegatables,
this is the one we buy as well as peas and sauerkraut. We like
to mix them all together. Corn is Jack's favorite canned food
while peas are mine.

Sometimes we eat canned vegetables as a break from fresh
vegetables because if we are ever in a situation where it is
necessary to eat something not quite as healthy as fresh
vegetables, it would not be such a shock to our systems.

Cucumbers
Protects the brain
Fights inflammation
Anitoxidant properties
Freshens breath
Manages stress
Beneficial for digestion
Maintains healthy weight
Supports heart health (136)

We both like cucumbers. I used to not like them and am glad
I changed my mind.

Dill Pickles
One cup equals 2 grams of fiber.
Low in calories
Essential vitamins and minerals
High in sodium (85)

We buy a big jar of big dill pickles, and I slice a plate or two of them to eat with our popcorn. This is a really good treat. I like to make a dill pickle and mustard sandwich. Even though I do not care for other pickles, I will eat them. I can tolerate bread and butter pickles, but not sweet ones or the relish made from them.

Garlic
Garlic contains allicin which has many potential medicinal properties. The sulphur in allicin is believed to provide the larger part of such health properties. Allicin is what gives garlic its offensive odor.
Garlic is from the onion family, is very nutritious, has few calories, and combats sickness including the common cold.
Reduces blood pressure
Improves cholesterol levels which may lower the risk of heart disease
Contains antioxidants that may prevent Alzeheimer's disease and dementia
May help you live longer
Athletic performance can be improved with garlic
Can help detoxify heavy metals in the body
Improves bone health
Easy to include in your diet and tastes absolutely delicious
Fights off viruses and bacterial infections
Helps maintain healthy cognitive function (35)

I cannot say enough good things about garlic. It has saved my life more than once. I cannot get enough of it.

I have read some where that eating too much garlic can cause your skin to bruise easily because it is such a good blood thinner. And that it is good to stop eating garlic, at least, two weeks before an operation due to the fact that the possiblity of hemorraging could occur.

We add it to salads and beans. I like to make a sandwich out of it with peanut butter and mustard.

Elephant garlic is good for you, but not as much as regular garlic. Some eat it because it does not have the odor. I have eaten it, but do not like it as much as the regular garlic.

Ginger
Soothes the stomach, muscle soreness, and cramps for women
Anti-viral and anti-carcinogenic
Helps with nausea and inflammation
Boosts the immune system
Helps with cholesterol
Improves cognitive functioning (19)

We like to add raw ginger to salads and a hot bowl of beans. It is really hot, but we like it.

Horseradish
Low in calories
Anti-inflammatory
Is a diuretic
Soothes nerves
Detoxifies
Has fiber, antioxidants, minerals, and vitamins such as vitamin C which helps alleviate viral infections by boosting immunity
Possesses a stimulant that increases appetite
Removes harmful free-radicals in order to protect against a variety of health issues such as cancer, inflammation, and infections (33)

Horseradish is great to add to a hot bowl of beans. No other spice or flavoring is needed. I made a mistake years ago and ate a teaspoonful by itself which resulted in a nosebleed.

Jack does not care for horseradish at all. If he eats things as spicy as this, he gets an allergic reaction.

Kale
Anti-inflammatory
Antioxidant
Supports the heart
Has detoxification properties
Good for healthy vision
Provides the brain development in infants
Aids in the prevention of cancer (74)

Kale and spinach are the only vegetables that have antioxidants values as high as berries. It tastes so good. We like it cooked or raw. It really tastes good to mix the raw and cooked together. Adding apple cider vinegar and olive oil gives it a really good taste.

Mushrooms
They are classified as vegetables, but are really fungus.
Antioxidant
Boost metabolism and the immune system
Contains Vitamin D
Good for the bladder
Helps prevent cancer
Reduces the risk of diabetes
Provides heart health
Great for weight management (72)

Even though I like mushrooms, I need to eat more than I do because they are good for osteoporosis due to the fact that they contain vitamin D. I like all mushrooms.

Jack does not like them as much as I do except for Portabello Mushrooms. When we go to the Veggie Grill in Los Angeles, we order a grilled Portabello Mushroom sandwich. It is so good. Portabellos have an unique taste.

All mushrooms are good in salad or eaten by themselves. I like to make a mushroom and mustard sandwich. Also, I dip them in mustard which is really good.

Onions
Provides the valuable prebiotic inulin and may prevent ulcers
Provides heart health
Lowers cholesterol
Decreases risk of coronary artery disease
Helps prevent peripheral vascular disease and stroke
Outer layers are most nutritious
Contain quercetin which is a powerful antioxidant with
anti-inflammatory properties
Contains sulfur compounds that have
anti-clotting properties (87)

We like to add onions to a pot of beans or soup as well as
salads. I like to eat them on a sandwich with mustard. They,
also, taste good boiled or microwaved. When I eat a lot of
them this way, my bowels really move tremendously.

They are good with fried potatoes. This is, basically, the only
fried food we eat.

Peas
Helps weight management
Good for stomach cancer preventation
Anti-aging, strong immune system, and high energy
Alzheimer's, arthritis, bronchitis, osteoporosis, candida,
and wrinkles
Provides blood sugar regulation
Promotes heart disease prevention
Beneficial for healthy bones
Reduces bad cholesterol
Prevents constipation
Healthy for environment regarding the soil (108)

Peas are my favorite canned food while corn is Jack's favorite.
We do not like the frozen ones. When we buy canned
vegatables, this is the one we buy as well as corn and
sauerkraut. We like to mix them together.

Sometimes we eat canned vegetables as a break from fresh vegetables because if we are ever in a situation where it is necessary to eat something not quite as healthy as fresh vegetables, it would not be such a shock to our systems.

Potatoes
80% water
Primarily carbohydrates
Small amounts of protein
Virtually no fat
High in fiber
Promotes colon health from the starch
Has many vitamins and minerals
Antioxidants which are mostly in the skin of the potato (89)

Almost everyday, we eat potatoes. They are not fattening like so many think. It is the things people add to the potatoes that are fattening such as butter and sour cream.

They taste really good when eaten raw, boiled, fried, or baked. Fried potatoes are, basically, the only fried food we eat. Sometimes we fry onions with the potatoes. Raw potatoes are really good with a little salt.

We put them in salads, soup, and a pot of beans. When used in soup or a pot of beans, they add thickening. We like to boil a big pot of potatoes and drink the broth. I like to put black pepper in my hot bowl of potato broth. Jack cannot do this because he has an allergy reaction to hot spices. The potatoes left from the broth are really good to eat cold.

Sauerkraut
Sauerkraut is an anti-inflammatory food that handles stress through "gut-brain" connection. It is a good source of antioxidants and dietary fiber, fights free radical damage, and is low in calories.

Sauerkraut has live "active probiotics" because it is a
fermented food. Probiotics are live bacteria and yeasts that
are good for your health, especially, your digestive system.
They are called "good" or "helpful" bacteria bcause they keep
your gut healthy. (20)
Protects cognitive health, brain disorders, and mental illness
Aids in preventing ulcerative colitis, irritable bowel
syndrome, digestive disorders such as leaky gut syndrome,
and the absorption of many nutrients
Handles stress and improves your mood such as disorders like
depression and anxiety
Provides cancer fighting antioxidants
Fights inflammation, allergies such as food allergies and
sensitivities, asthma, and a variety of auto-immune diseases
Helps with hormonal imbalances
Good for metabolic conditions such as diabetes
Beneficial for weight maintenance such as obesity and
weight gain
Detoxifies the body (21)

When we buy canned vegatables, this is the one we buy as
well as peas and corn. We like to mix them together.
It is, also, good to eat by itself. It is healthier to buy it in a jar
instead of a can.

Sometimes we eat canned vegetables as a break from fresh
vegetables because if we are ever in a situation where it is
necessary to eat something not quite as healthy as fresh
vegetables, it would not be such a shock to our systems.

Spinach
Anti-inflammatory support
Regulates hunger and blood sugar levels
Good for cancer prevention
Reduces inflammation in the digestive tract (75)
Low in carbs – They are only found in fiber.

Contains many vitamins and minerals
Provides for oxidative stress
Regulates blood pressure levels
Improves eye health (76)

Spinach and kale are the only vegetables that have
antioxidants values as high as berries. Spinach is really good
for the bowels.

Both of us really like it a lot. Adding apple cider vinegar to
spinach is really good as well as apple cider vinegar and olive
oil.

GRAINS
Lowers risk of Type 2 diabetes
Contains fiber to help prevent certain cancers
Prevents heart failure
High antioxidant
Prevents artherosclerosis, ischemic stroke, obesity, asthma, and
stroke
Reduces inflammation
Lowers risk of colorectal cancer
Aids in healthier blood pressure levels
Beneficial for less gum disease and tooth loss (61)

We like to put grains in a salad, a hot bowl of beans, or eat
them by themself. Grains and beans combined creates a
complete protein. Soybeans are the only beans that are a
complete protein without adding grains.

I usually cook one type of grain at a time. But sometimes I
cook a variety of grains together. When they are done, I add
water as well as oatmeal and let it cook for just a few minutes
more. I let it cool so it will pack together. This mixture taste
like a breakfast food.

Couscous
Protein – one cup contains 6 grams and 12% of the daily
required amount of protein
Contains fiber
Has essential vitamins and trace minerals (60)

This is one food that you do not have to chew because it is so
fine. It tastes good by itself or added to a hot bowl of beans.
Adding soy sauce or Bragg's Amino Acids is really good, too.

Oatmeal
Contains many vitamins and minerals,
High in fiber
Antioxidants
Helps with weight loss because it is so filling
Gluten free
Improves blood sugar
Lowers cholesterol
Helps with skin care
Aids in constipation
Good for childhood asthma (54)

Oatmeal is best for you if left overnight in water to ferment and
provide a natural bacteria. I throw a handfull of uncooked
oatmeal in a hot bowl of beans or tomato juice.

When I cook a variety of grains together, after they are done, I
add water as well as oatmeal to the mixture and let it cool so it
will pack together. This tastes like a breakfast food.

Popcorn
Whole grain
High in nutrients
Healthy low-calorie snack
Antioxidants
Protects against free-radicals

High in fiber
Vitamins
Minerals

How To Make Healthy Popcorn – (Air-Popped
is best)
3 Tablespoon of olive oil or coconut oil,
½ Cup of kernels,
Onion powder or ½ teaspoon salt,
Sprinkle a tablespoon or so of nutritional yeast (147)

Jack makes popcorn for us this way. It is really good. He uses
canola oil, nutritional yeast, onion powder, and/or salt.

Quiona
High in protein
Gluten free
Great source of fiber
Provides heart health
Antioxidant
Nutritious superfood which helps with such aliments like leg
cramps, muscle pain, insomnia, and anxiety
Contains iron
Good for weight loss
Helps prevent cancer
Reduces risk of diabetes
Fights diseases such as cardiovascuar disease
Contains all the necessary amino-acids for good health (56)

Just a little quiona fills us up. We eat it by itself or add it to a
hot bowl of beans. When we add soy sauce or Bragg's Amino
Acids it is really good. We, also, like to eat it plain. It has a
really good taste.

RICE
Brown Rice
Rich in Seleium
Reduces risk of cancer, heart disease, and arthritis
High in manganese
Helps the body synthesize fats
Benefits the nervous and reproductive systems
Rich in naturally occuring oils
Helps normalize cholesterol levels
Promotes weight loss – makes you feel fuller
High in fiber
Aids with bowel function
Prevents colon cancer
Is a whole grain
Reduces risk of arerial plaque, heart disease, and
high cholesterol
Rich in anti-oxidants
Stabilizes blood sugar
Good to treat candida infections (58)

We eat brown rice by itself or add soy sauce or Bragg's Amino
Acids. It is good when added to a hot bowl of beans. We like
to eat it with a stir-fry.

It is good to limit eating brown rice because the bran contains a
small amount of arsenic. But it is better for you than white rice
because the bran, which is healthy for you even though it
contains a small amount of asenic, has been removed from
white rice. It is better to limit oneself to either one. But both
are better for you than the average American diet.

Although white rice is not as nutritious as the brown, we have
cooked both of them together.

White Rice
It is not as healthy as brown rice because the bran is removed.
But the bran contains arsenic; so it is better to limit oneself to
either kind. Even though white rice is not as healthy as brown

rice, it is a better alternative to the average American diet (140)

Although white rice is not as nutritious as the brown, we have cooked both of them together.

Wheat Germ
Good for the immune system
Beneficial for cardioascular health
Risk of coronary heart diseases is lessened
Cancer prevention
Has anti-aging properties
Aids in cellular metabolism
Maintains healthy muscles which aids in athletic performance, helping to improve stamina performance
Reduces risk of diabetes
Helps with pregnancy
Gluten free

We add wheat germ to salads and a hot bowl of beans.

JUICE
Cranberry, grape, and orange juice give me a heartburn if I drink them too fast. But this has no such effect on Jack.

Cranberry Juice
Helps to prevent cancer, lung inflammation, heart diseases caused by plaque, and urinary tract infection as well as an aid to cure it
Provides anti-tumor effects
Beneficial for cardiovascular health
Avoids respiratory infections
Cures colds and sore throats
Good for obesity, scurry, and stomach disorders such as peptic ulcers
Prevents kidney stones; but you should not take it if you already have kidney stones
Has anti-aging benefits

Strengthens the immune system, bones, and teeth as well as preventing tooth decay
Relieves stress
If you are allergic to aspirin or taking blood thinners such as Warfarin, do not use cranberry juice. (24)

We drink a shot of pure cranberry juice every other day or so. It really taste bad and curls your toes.

Ocean Spray Cranberyy Juice gave me a heartburn when I used to drink it; but the pure cranberry juice does not. Jack does not get a heartburn from the Ocean Spray.

My cousin Dixie used to mix half Ocean Spray and half of the pure together. It tasted good, but we prefer not to consume the sugar in the Ocean Spray.

Grape Juice
Grape juice has antioxidants that fight harmful free radicals in your body that can damage cells and cause disease. Some of its benefits include fighting against blood clots as well as an excellent brain booster.
Is fat and cholesterol free
Contains very low in sodium
An excellent source of vitamin C
Good source of managanese
Has no added sugar
It is good for the brain (25)

Grape juice is really heavy. If I drink it too quickly, I get a heartburn. It does not bother Jack this way.

Orange Juice
Oranges have fiber, but orange juice does not; so for the complete benefit of oranges, eat the whole orange, instead of just the juice.
Boosts immune system

Beneficial in cancer prevention
Provides detoxifying properties
Good for blood pressure
Balances cholesterol
Reduces risk of cardiovascular disease and macular
degeneration
Rich in antioxidant and anti-inflammatory properties
Aids in improving blood circulation and creation of red
blood cells (28)

I cannot drink orange juice very quickly or I get heartburn. It
does not bother Jack this way. He likes it better than me.

Tomato Juice
Packed with vitamins
Lowers cholesterol
Detoxifies the body
Prevents various diseases such as cancer
Aids in weight loss
Improves skin tone
Good for the hair (37)

Tomato juice is my favorite juice. It helps curb our appetites.
I like it cold or heated. Jack only likes it heated.

We drink a warm cup when we are hungry and do not want to
eat yet. It is, also, satisfying to heat up a cup of tomato juice
before we eat when feeling that our bodies are not ready for
solid food even though we are hungry. It reminds me of
tomato soup. At times, the juice is so thick that I add water or
vegetable broth to a cup before heating it.

It is healthy to add oil as well as seeds to a hot cup. Sometimes
I add olive oil, sunflower seeds, or rasins. When I add rasins, it
really fills me up.

I heat a cup at work and add two teaspoons of oatmeal as well as one teaspoon of flaxseed for my lunch if I am hungry. It is just enough to fill me up without making me feel too full while I am working.

LECITHIN
Treats conditions of the brain, like Alzheimer's and other forms of dementia – anxiety and some types of depression
Reduces symptoms associated with manic-depressive disorder, like hallucinations, delusions, and jumbled speech
Taken for head injuries and memory impairment due to aging
Moistures the skin
Beneficial for liver and gallbladder disease, eczema, and high cholesterol (45)
Is essential for proper functioning of the nervous system (46)

Lecithin tastes awful, but it is so good for you. We usually take a tablespoon every other day. It is really thick and sticks to roof of your mouth.

MILK
Almond Milk
Manages weight
Impacts blood sugar
Keeps heart healthy, skin glowing, and digestion in check
Contributes to muscles strength and healing as well as keeps bones strong
Better than cow's milk because it does not contain lactose or require refrigeration
Easy to make (30)
Soy Milk
Improves lipid blood profile
Strengthens blood vessel integrity
Promotes weight loss
Beneficial in preventing prostate cancer, post menopausal syndrome, and osteoporosis (29)

Although soy milk is good for you, almond milk is healthier.
I like to drink either one when I am hungry and do not want to
eat.   Jack's favorite is vanilla. My favorite is chocolate.

NUTS
Are considered a fruit
Among the healthiest foods you can eat
Great source of many nutrients
Loaded with antioxidants
Helps lose weight
Lower in cholesterol and triglycerides
Beneficial for Type 2 diabetes
Helps reduce inflammation
High in fiber
Reduces risk for heart attack
Delicious, versatile, and widely available (145)

We mix a lot of nuts together as a trail-mix. Dr. Oz said that
nuts are more nutritious if you soak them overnight. I think I
get more nutrition from them this way because I can chew
them better.

Almond Butter
Has many vitamins, minerals, and protein
Provides high amounts of essential fatty acids as well as
Omega-3 fatty acids
Contains unsaturated fat which is a healthy fat
Lowers cholesterol (109)

Peanut Butter
Aids with weight loss
Packed with nutrition
Contains the antioxidant vitamin E
Provides good fat which is a
healthy monounsaturated fat
Boosts immune system
Fights diabetes (112)

When I want just a snack, I will get a tablespoon of either one and eat it that way. We like both of these. almond butter is really filling. At Smith's grocery in Las Vegas, we grind our own almond and peanut butter. It is pure with no added oils and is not hydrogenated.

Almonds
Maintains dental and bone health
Contains cholesterol
Heart health such as preventing heart disease and heart attacks
Supports brain health such as Alzheimer's
Promotes skin health
Controls blood sugar levels and prevents diabetes
Helps with weight loss – prevents overeating
Healthy metabolism
Increases nutrient absorption and digestive health
Beneficial to fight cancer, inflammation, and
free radicals (110)

I have studied that 10-12 almonds are good for you a day. They contain Laetrile which has been known to cure cancer. We really like them.

Brazil Nuts
If you overdose on them, they can damage your DNA. Two to four nuts a day is good. (116)
High selenium content might produce liver and kidney toxcidity. Only eat four a month (117)
Great for the immune system
Boost metabolism
Protects against cancer
Aids in sexual performance
Improves overall health (116)

Brazil nuts are shaped like a toe. We really do not like these nuts but eat them.

Cashews
Fights heart disease
Helps prevent gallstones
Weight loss and maintenance
Maintains bone health
Prevents migraines and cancers such as colon, prostate,
and liver
Supports healthy brain function
Lowers risk for diabetes
Provides healthy skin (138)

We both really like cashews a lot.

Hazelnuts
High in fiber
Promotes heart health
Lowers cholesterol
Manages diabetes
Filled with antioxidants
Vitamin E – that helps with aging and disease by
reducing inflammation
Beneficial to the brain - Prevents and treats Alzheimer's as
well as Parkinson's
Helps prevent cancer
Combats obesity
Boosts metabolism
Improves digestion
Contributes to healthy skin and hair (115)

Hazelnuts are really hard in texture and do not tastes very
good. They are easier to eat if you soak them overnight. We
do not really care for them.

Macadamia Nuts
High in fiber
Contains a cardio-protective trace element
Packed with many health-benefiting nutrients, vitamims,
and minerals
Rich source of monounsaturated fatty acids, like oleic acid
that helps lower blood pressure
Rich source of energy (114)

Macadamia nuts have an excellent, buttery, and rich taste. We
really like them a lot.

Peanuts
Peanuts are legumes.
Provide heart healthy monounsaturated fats
Has as many antioxidants comparable to fruits
Contains oleic acid which is the healthy fat
Reduces risk of stroke, gallstones, and colon cancer
Helps prevent Alzheimer's and age-related cognitive decline
Good for weight loss (111)

Peanuts are always good and an old stand-by. They are one of
our favorites.

Pecans
Has high levels of monounsaturated fats like oleic acid
Great for cardiovascular health
Promotes digestive health
Provides for weight loss
Contains many vitamins and minerals
Reduces risk of cancer
Good for bone and teeth health
Has anti-inflammatory benefits that fight free radicals
Strengthens immune system
Prevents skin problems
Helps maintain clean complexion
Prevents hair loss
Beneficial for anti-aging benefits (120)

Pecans really tastes good. We like them.

Walnuts
One-fourth cup provides100% of the daily recommended
requirement of plant Omega-3 fats.
Is heart health
Provides cancer-fighting properties
Contains protein
High in fiber
Great for weight control
Has many vitamins and minerals
Contains plant steroids and healthy fats
Improves reproducive health in men
Beneficial for diabetes
Provides a rare and powerful antioxdant
90% of antioxidants are in the skin of walnuts
Fights against chemically induced liver damage (113)

Walnuts have a rich, good taste. We like them.

OIL
Canola Oil
It is considered healthy because it is low in saturated fats. Like
olive oil, it is high in monosaturated fat
Reduces blood pressure and cholesterol
Helps prevent heart disease
Provides Omega-3 and fatty acids (71)

When we fry foods such as potatoes and stir-fry we use canola
oil. We like to put it on baked potatoes and corn on the cob.
It is, also, good in a salad. Jack uses it when he makes
popcorn for us.

Coconut Oil

Helps memory and cognitive function
Aids in weight loss
Is a healthy butter and cooking oil replacement
Speeds up the metabolism and increases energy
Reduces constipation
Boosts your immune system
Brings emotional balance
Makes the skin look and feel healthy and beautiful (17)

When we add coconut oil to a salad or a hot bowl of beans, we do not need any other spices or flavorings. We put a tablespoon of it and a little turmeric in a cup of coffee which has been said will prevent Alzheimer's.

We do Oil Pulling which is a tablespoon of coconut oil used to swish around in your mouth for, at least, 15-20 minutes, spit it out, rinse your mouth out, and then brush your teeth. When you spit it out, do not spit it down the drain because it can clog the drains up. Oil Pulling helps if I am starting to get a toothache.

Jack's filling fell out. It could have been from the Oil Pulling because sometimes that is a result from using it.

Olive Oil

Fights inflammation, cancer, coronary heart disease, diabetes, and degenerative nerve diseases
Aids in preventing Alzheimer's
Beneficial in preventing coronary artery disease and strokes
Contains Omega-6, antioxidants, vitamins, and phyto-sterois
Less saturated than most oils
Rich in mono-unsaturated fatty oils
Lowers LBL (bad cholesterol)
Increases HDL (good cholesterol)
Reduces risk of heart disease

Inhibits cholesterol absorption
High in calories
Rich in vitamin E and vitamin K
Provides oxygen free radials
Increases bone mass (44)

Olive oil and apple cider vinegar is our salad dressing. I like
to put a teaspoon in a hot cup of tomato juice.

SEEDS
Chia
Provides many nutrients and few calories
Loaded with antioxidants
Almost all the carbs are fiber
High in protein
Good to lose weight because of the high fiber and
protein content
High in Omega-3 fatty acids
Improves certain blood markers which should lower the risk of
heart disease and Type 2 diabetes
Provides bone nutrients
Improves exercise performance as much as a
sports drink
Easy to incorporate in your diet (55)

We add chia to a salad or a hot bowl of beans. It is impossible
to chew them because they are so small and hard. We really
could not say what they taste like. But they are good for us; so
we consume them.

Flaxseed
High in fiber
Low in carbs
Provides healthy skin and hair
Good for weight loss
Lowers cholesterol

Gluten free
High in antioxidants and Omega-3 fatty acids
Good for digestive health
Helps with cancer prevention
Beneficial for menopausal symtoms (57)

We add flaxseeds to a salad or a hot bowl of beans. I, also, like
to add it to a hot cup of tomato juice. This fills me up.

Hemp Seeds
Are nutritious
Reduces the risk of heart attack
Benefits skin disorders
Great source of plant-based protein
Reduces symtoms of PMS and menopause
Aids digestion (135)

Hemp seeds tastes good to eat raw by itself; but we add it to a
salad or a hot bowl of beans.

Millet
Millet is a seed; but it is often considered a grain
Has heart-protective properties
Aids in the development and repair of body tissures
Lowers risk of Type 2 dibetes
Helps prevent gallstones
Contains fiber to help prevent breast cancer
Helps with childhood asthma
Health-preventing activity equal to or even higher than
vegetables and fruits
Prevents heart disease and heart failure
Provides cardiocascular benefits for
postmenopausal women
High in antioxidants (59)

Millet is a seed we add to a salad or a hot bowl of beans. It taste good when we eat it cooked by itself and maybe add a little soy sauce or Bragg's Amino Acids. We have always thought of it as a grain.

Pumpkin Seeds
Good for the liver, heart, and prostate
Provides zinc for immune support
Contains plant-based Omega-3 fat
Aids with anti-diabetic effects
Beneficial for postmenopausal women
Has tryptohan for restful health (121)

Pumpkin seeds are a great snack and very filling. We include them in a trail-mix with our nuts.

Sunflower Seeds
Promotes cardiovascular health and healthy cholesterol
Great for the systems of nerves, immune, muscle, skeleton, and respiratory.
Reduces PMS tension
Good for heart health
Provides a healthy mood
Contains selenium: a powerful antioxidant great for thyroid health and has the ability to encourage DNA repair in damaged cells
Reduces redness and swelling in the body (122)

If I soak sunflower seeds overnight, they are easier to eat. It is healthy to put them in a cup of heated tomato juice. We include them in a trail-mix with our nuts.

SALSA
Four calories in one tablespoon
Povides good health, lycopene, and vitamins (131), (132)

Not only do we use salsa for tortilla chips, it really tastes good as a dip for vegetables and fruit. When we eat a lot, our bowels move really good the next day.

SPAGHETTI

Contains carbs which provide energy as well as many nutrients such as many vitamins and minerals. One great benefit is fiber, especially, in whole grain and whole wheat pasta. (141)

It is quite difficult for us to find spaghetti we can eat. Even though the package might say "vegan", if it says that it was "processed in a facility that processes milk and eggs", we will not eat it due to the fact that we do not eat anything relating to the death of animals. Jack likes it better than me. It stops my bowels up if I eat too much.

SPAGHETTI SAUCE

High in fiber as well as sodium
Lowers cholesterol
Provides many vitamins
Contains calories from sugar
Provides lycopene (128)

Not only do we use spaghetti sauce on spaghetti, we like to use it as a dip for vegetables and fruits.

SPICES
Black Pepper
Improves digestion
Promotes intestinal health (62)

I really like black pepper a lot and cannot get enough of it. It really tastes good when I sprinkle it on most of my food. Jack cannot eat it because he gets an allergic reaction; but it does not bother him if it is cooked into food. He likes to add it to fried potatoes along with salt.

Cayenne Pepper
Contains properties of anti-cold and flu agent, anti-allergen, anti-fungal, anti-redness, and anti-bacterial
Produces salica
Is a pain reliever
Possible anti-cancer agent
Promotes heart health
Topical remedy for toothache (42)
One of the major benefits of cayenne pepper is the positive effect it has on the digestive system.
Beneficial for migraine pain
Prevents blood clots
Provides detox support
Relieves joint and nerve pain
Supports weight loss
Works as an anti-irritant
Boosts metabolism (43)

I add this to a salad or a hot bowl of beans. Jack cannot do this because he has an allergic reaction to hot spices.

Cumin
Controls diabetes
Aids digestion
Contains essential minerals (63)

Cumin can make any pot of beans taste like chilli.

One time when I was living in Kansas City, Jack came to see me. The only thing we ate all week was lentils with cumin cooked in it. We noticed that Jack's bald spots were starting to grow thin pieces of hair. Maybe he should try eating only lentils with cumin for awhile and maybe get a new crop of hair. (HA!)

Onion Power
Is a dietary fiber
Provides many vitamins and minerals such as Vitamin C
and calcium (66)

Onion Powder is a very good replacement for salt in many
ways. Sometimes Jack uses this instead of salt in popcorn
with canola oil. Or he might use salt and onion powder
together with the canola oil.

Par D' Arco
Strengthens the immune system
Good for inflammation
Treatment for a wide variety of health issues such as viruses,
candida and other fungus, skin disorders such as eczema,
herpes, and more, polio, influenza, arthritis, diabetes,
parasites, bacteria, cancer, veneral diseases, and
rheumaic disorders. Helps prevent and cure cancer (41)

We add this to a salad or a hot bowl of beans. It has a horrible
taste, but is so good for us.

Salt
1,500 mg of sodium amounts to 0.75 teaspoon 3.75 grams
recommended per day (64)
Salt is good because it contains iodine; but seaweed is the best
source and has much less sodium than salt. It offers many
other health benefits.
Gargling with salt may help prevent the common cold.
Too much salt cause many illnesses such as: kidney stones,
dry eye disease, obesity, heart disease, stroke, and high
blood pressure. (65)

I use a few sprinkles of salt every other day and sometimes
everyday. The Iodine in the salt is good for you. Even though
sea salt is the best, we just use the regular.

In the past, I have used the 'false salt' because if I eat too much
regular salt, I get a pain in my chest. But if cook with
it, I have no problems.

Now I just use the regular because I feel that I need the Iodine.
And the 'false salt' is just chemicals put together to taste like
regular salt. Plus, I always use too much of the 'false salt'
while I do not with the regular. Salt has no negative effect on
Jack.

Jack uses salt when he fries potatoes and sometimes with the
popcorn he makes. Sometimes he uses salt and onion
powder together with canola oil when he pops popcorn.

Turmeric
Overall decrease of cancer risk
Provides cardiovascular benefits
Helps with chronic digestive health problems including
Chron's disease and ulcerative colitis as well as inflammatory
bowel diseases
Contains Omega acids and curcumia which is an important
health-supportive substance
Beneficial to the nerve system
Potential help with Alzeheimer's
Regulates inflammation, oxidation, cell signaling, blood sugar
levels, blood fat levels, and brain levels of the Omega-3 fatty
acid called DHA (40)

A guy on the Dr. Oz Show said that turmeric and coconut oil
with a cup of coffee helps to ward-off Alzheimer's. We drink
a cup of this almost everyday. Sometimes we add it to a salad
and a hot bowl of beans. It has a horrible taste but is so good
for us.

TEA
When I take tea to work, I make it and let it set overnight.
Then I pour it in a plastic container and drink it at work.

Jack likes the teas that have a fruit flavor and the apple cinnamon as well as the ones listed below. Although these are quite healthy, I do not care for them at all. I just drink the ones listed below.

Chai Tea
Contains antioxidants that prevent disease, neutralizes free radicals
Reduces risk of cancer, strokes, heart attacks, high cholesterol, and tooth decay
Has no calories, fat, carbohydrates, protein, or vitamins
Contains caffeine
Decreases risk of developing kidney stones and osteoporosis (126)

This is my favorite tea. It is very filling. I like to take it to work to curb my appetite because I do not like to eat much while I am working. Jack does not care for it.

Green Tea
Healthiest beverage on the planet
Contains bioactive compounds that improve health such as being loaded with antioxdants and nutrients that have powerful effects on the body
Improves physical performance
Contains compounds that improve brain function, makes you smarter, and protects your brain in old age which helps lower the risk of Alzheimer's and Parkinson's
Kills bacteria, which improves dental health and lowers risk of infections
Lowers risk of Type 2 diabetes
Helps fight heart disease and reduces risk of cardiovascular disease
Helps you lose weight by fighting obesity
Decreases risk of dying and helps you live longer
Helps avoid strokes (16), (123)

Green tea is the most healthiest of all teas. I really do not like it; but I drink it because it is so healthy. I have to drink it slowly throughout the day because it makes me so nauseated. When I use a green tea and another kind together, it tastes so much better and does not nauseate me.

Mint Medley Tea
Mint has one of the highest antioxidant capabilities of any food.
Beneficial for irritable bowel syndrome, indigestion, and gas
Provides for pain relief
Aids in curing gastric ulcers
Good for oral health and skin
Provides many vitamins and minerals
Beneficial health for allergies
Great when breast feeding
Helps relieves the common cold (125)

Peppermint Tea
Is considered a stomach healer that assists with digestion such as irritable bowel syndrome, nausea, stomach aches, diarrhea, and constipation.
Relieves stress
Boosts immune system
Reduces bad breath
Beneficial for many health issues such as fever and cough (124)

These teas give a soothing type of feeling. We both like them very much. These are some of Jack's favorites. Even though I like them, he likes them better than I do.

Smooth Move
Relieves constipaiton, generally, produces a bowel movement
within 6-12 hours (127)

Smooth Move is great for the bowels. But make sure a
restroom is nearby the next day. It creates a cramping
sensation when the bowels are moving, but the pain is
well-worth it.

The Smooth Move they made years ago was better than
today's even though it is the same brand. But today's Smooth
Move is still quite effective. It has kind of a licorce flavor.

TOFU
Tofu does a better job of reducing the risk of stomach cancer
than any other soy, in general.
Tofu is made from soybeans.
Prevents Type 2 diabetes and cancer (31)
Excellent source of amino acids, iron, calcium, and many
other micro-nutrients
Has 8 essential amino-acids
Similar to the female hormone estrogen
Lowers cholesterol, preventing heart disease, and aiding in
cardiovascular health (32)

We eat tofu in different ways including just plain. Although
we prefer the extra firm, we will eat it in any form. It is good
to put in salads, a hot bowl of beans, soup, and just cut in
pieces with soy sauce.

Jack makes stir-fries and adds tofu to it. I have fried it and
scrambled it up. Then added different spices. I added
turmeric to give it a yellow flavor. This combination resulted
in it tasting like scrambled eggs.

VINEGAR
Apple Cider Vinegar
Skip coffee and have a tablespoon of vinegar with some water or orange juice to increase energy levels for the day.
Solves an upset stomach
Eliminates hiccups
Sore throat cure
Reduces cholesterol and contains no dietary cholesterol
Stops indigestion
Clears nose from constipation and stuffiness
Helps to lose weight
Beneficial for dry scalp
Aid to blemishes on your face
Prevents harsh leg cramps at night
Stops chronic bad breath
Eliminates bruising on the skin
Protective for the heart
Prevents cancer
Alleviates sunburn pain
Body-fat lowering, reduces body mass index, waist circumference, and triglyceride levels
Can erode the teeth
Contains no fat protein (18), (69)

There are so many things that occur as a result of using apple cider vinegar. We use it almost everyday either straight or with food. Jack and I have read, and believe, that apple cider vinegar is a 'cure-all'.

Bragg's Apple Cider Vinegar
Contains the Mother of Vinegar which occurs naturally as a strand-like enzymes of connected protein molecules. (133)
Contains iron and B-vitamins
High in prebiotics
Good source of phenolin compounds that help prevent disease, one of these is galllic acid which is, also, found in tea and grapes. (134)

Heinz Apple Cider Vinegar
Has no calories, fat, carbs, or protein (68)
Is an appetite suppressant – can lose weight
Prevents fat accummulation
Controls blood sugar
Beneficial impact on insulin secretion
Detoxifies the body (69)

We usually buy Heinz Apple Cider Vinegar even though
Bragg's Apple Cider Vinegar with The Mother is the
healthiest. It has to be refrigerated while Heinz does not.

If we have a heartburn, it is great to use. Just a capfull usually
takes it away. It really burns the throat at the beginning, but it
is worth the relief it ends up giving.

Apple cider vinegar is great to lose weight because it curbs
your appetite. It can, also cure, symtoms of an ulcer. Years
ago, Jack weighed over 200 pounds and was developing
symtoms of an ulcer. I gave him a book to read about apple
cider vinegar.

He started taking a capfull of Heinz Apple Cider Vinegar
throughout the day and even carried a bottle in his car; so he
could take it often. Jack lost the weight he wanted and the
ulcer symtoms disappeared.

WATER
Distilled And Purified
The only difference between distilled and purified water is
that distilled water goes through distillation while purified
goes through other processes such as reverse osmosis, ion
exchange, ozonation, sand filtration, etc. But distilled water is
actually purified water; the process of distillation is one of the
technologies used to purify water. (148)

We drink only distilled water or purified. But we still cook, make coffee, and bathe with regular water because I feel that it is, at least, sterilized when using it this way. We refill our gallon jugs at water machines found at various places such as grocery stores, gas stations, and Wal-Mart.

It is best to not drink water with a meal because the natural enzymes in the salva are not as effective.

I drink it when I eat peanuts or raw carrots because these foods make me thristy and cause me to drink a lot of water.

YEAST
Brewer's Yeast
Has vitamin B12
Contains B-complex vitamins as well as chromium, a trace amino acid that regulates blood sugar
Is a by-product of beer-making

Nutritional Yeast
Nutrional yeast is grown on sugar beets, sugar beet molasses, or sugar cane molasses
Contains protein
Has B vitamins such as B12 which is vital to vegans
Provides all the 9 essential amino acids
Good for candida infection, chronic acne, loss of appetite, diarrhea, immune system stimulation, easily digested, and athletes use it frequently (52)

Nutritional Yeast has a very good flavor. We add it to salads, a hot bowl of beans, and popcorn.

We do not use Brewer's Yeast. Years ago I used to use it. That was before I knew about Nutritional Yeast.

TERMS
Acrylamide
Antioxidants
Enzymes
Free-Radicals
Lycopene
Oxidative Stress
Probiotics
Sulfur
Tannins
Quercetin

EXPLANTIONS OF TERMS
Acrylamide
Acrylamide is a chemical used in many industrial processes.
Also, found in many foods such as potato chips, french fries,
and olives. It is a probable cause of human carcinogen. (104)

Antioxidants
Antioxidants are powerful substances, such as beta-carotene
and vitamin C, that come, mostly, from fresh fruits
and vegetables. They prohibit and prevent the oxidation of
other molecules in the body such as reactions presented by
oxygen, and peroxides while fighting against free radicals
that enter your body. (95), (96)

Enzymes
Enzymes are substances produced by the body cells that helps
bring about or speeds up bodily chemical activities (as in
digestion of food) without being destroyed in
this process (118)
Enzymes are the sparks that start the essential chemical
reactions our bodies need to live. They are necessary for
digesting food, stimulating the brain, providing cellular
energy, and repairing tissues. All enzymes are protein, but not
all proteins are enzymes. (119)

Free Radicals

Antioxidants are substances whose jobs are to clean up free radicals, just like fiber cleans up waste in the cells. (97)
Free radicals are formed as a result of diet, stress, smoking, alcohol, exposure to sunlight, drugs, and pollutants. The most common is oxygen breathing. (98)

Lyopene

Tomatoes and tomato products contain lyopene.
Lyopene is more effective for you by heating tomato juice with oil.
Good for immune system
Possesses antioxidants that fight free radicals
Helps prevent cancer (129)
Best to eat with avocadoes, oil, and seeds
One of the most powerful antioxidants in the world
Heal your body from damage from pesticides
Great for the eyes like with macular degeneration
Good for the nerves and alleviates neuropathic pain
Benefits the brain as with Alzheimer's
Prevents high blood pressure and heart disease
Helps the bones become strong
Provides healing and prevention of vaginal
yeast infections (130)

Oxidative Stress

Is an inbalance between the production of free radicals and the ability of the body to conteract or detoxify their harmful effects through neutralization by antioxidants. (99)

Probiotics

Probiotics are live bacteria and yeasts that are good for your health, especially, your digestive system. They are 'good' bacteria because they help keep your gut healthy. (139)

Quercetin

Antioxidant found in plant foods
Improves endurance
Fights free radical damage
Anti-inflammatory
Prevents cancer
Helps aging process
Great for the immune system
Lowers inflammation which is the root cause of most diseases
Fights allergies
Lowers cholesterol
Fights pain
Good for skin health
Is in many plant foods and green tea (107)

Sulfur

Sulfur is used in the formation of amino acids, protein, and oils. It activates certain enzymes and provides many essential vitamins. It is a structural component of two of the 21 amino acids that form protein. (81)

Tannins

Tannins are a broad class of compounds that is present in tea, coffee, red wine, cocoa, chocolate, and some herbal preparations, grapes, and certain fruits like blackberries and cranberries. (93)
The astringent tannin is effective in oral hygiene when used as a gargle or mouthwash.
The leaves are good for tea.
Alleviates hemorroids and soothes the efects of diarreha.
Helps cure cancers of the GI tract, like colon cancer
Reduces age-related conditions, such as Alzeheimer's and dementia
Helps with mild inflammation of the gums and throat
Provides lots of vitamin k; so they are very effective in helping with blood clots as well as menstruation

Improves athletic performance
Reduces risk of many diseases
Good for overall health (94)

Daily Required Nutritional Grams For The Average Adult Based On A 2000 Calorie Diet

Grains: 9 grams daily (13)
Fats: 44 to 78 grams daily (12)
Fruits: 150 grams of fresh fruit or 50 grams of dried
fruit daily   (14)
Protein: 50 grams for a man and 46 grams for a woman. (4)
Vegetables: 75 grams daily (14)

REFERENCES

11 Health Benefits Of Beans/Huffington Post
www.huffingtonpost.com/2012/08/26 beans – health – benefits _ n _ 1792504.html
(1)

Health Benefits Of Beans
www.foods – healing – power.com/health – health -benefits – of – beans (2)

healthyeating.sfgate.com/types – beans – highest – amount –
protein – 68.35.html (3)

http//authority.nutrition.com//how – much – protein – per – day (4)

Profile Of Beans/HealthyEating
healthyeatingsfgatecom/amino – acids – profile – beans – 4952.html Amino Acid
(5)

http://consumer healthyday.com/-/antioxidants../benefits-beans-top-best-
antioxidants (6)

What Are The Benefits Of Combining Beans And Grains?
healthyeating.sfgate.com > Nutrition > Amino-Acids (7)

Soy Connection By The United Soybean Board
www.soybeanconnection.com/soyfoods/nutritional_composition.php (8)

What Are Amino Acids?/aminoacid-studies.com
www.aminoacid-studies.com > Amino-Acids (9)

WHAT IS THE "POOR MAN'S MEAT?" - CHELSEA GREEN PUBLISHING
www.chelseagreen.com/what-is-the-poor-man's-meat/ (10)

Top Foods To Lower Blood Pressure – GB Health Watch
www.gbhealthwatch.com/Did-you-know-top-foods-to-lower-blood-pressure.php
(11)

www.healtheating.sfgate.com > Diet > Eat (12)

www.usda.gov/factbook/chapter2.htm (13)

www.abs.gov.au/ausstots/abs@.nsf/Lookup/bysubject/4338.0-2011-13 (14)

BENEFITSOF BRAGG LIQUID SOY SEASONING|LIVESTRONG.COM
www.livestrong.com > Food and Drink (15)

9 BENEFITS OF GREEN TEA-healthremediesjournal.com
www.healthremediesjournal.com/ (16)

COCONUT OIL.NUTRITION FACTS AND HEALTHY BENEFITS-
NUTRITION AND YOU
www.nutrition-and-you.com/coconut-oil.html (17)

VINEGAR-WHAT IS THE NUTRITIONAL VALUE OF
VINEGAR?|LIVESTRONG.COM
www.livestrong/com > Food and Drink (18)

Top 9 Benefits of Ginger – Health Remedies Journal
www.healthremediesjournalcom/top-9-benefits-of-ginger/ (19)

WHAT ARE PROBIOTICS? BENEFITS. SUPPLEMENTS. FOODS. AND
MORE-WEB MD
www.webmd.com/digestive-disorders/features/what-are-probiotics (20)

7 BENEFITS OF SAUERKRAUT. PLUS HOW TO MAKE YOUR OWN-DR.
AXE
https:/drxe.com/sauerkraut (21)

THE BENEFITS OF YELLOW MUSTARD/LIVESTRONG.COM
www.livestrong.com > Food and Drink (22)

TOMATO KETCHUP-7 SURPRISING HEALTHBENEFITS YOU MUST READ
http://www.cookingdetectives.com > Food and Drinks > Vegetable (23)

HEALTH BENEFITS OF CRANBERRY JUICE/ORGANIC FACTS
http://www.organicfacts.net/health-benefits/fruit/health-benefits-of-cranberry-
juice.html (24)

GRAPEJUICE (100%)-NUTRITION-SELECTION-STORAGE-FRUITS AND
VEGGIES ...
www.fruitsand veggiesmoremattersorg >... > Fruit Nutrition (25)

HEALTH BENEFITS OF FRUIT – FRUITS AND VEGGIES MORE
MATTERS.ORG
www.fruit and veggiesmorematters.org (26)

http://authoritynutrition.com/12-proven-benefits-of-avocado/
(27)

https://www.organicfacts.net > fruits (28)

6 BENEFITS OF SOY MILK/NUTRITION/HEALTHY EATING FIT DAY
www.fitday.com/fitness-articles/nutrition/healthy.../6-health-benefits-of-soy-
milk.html (29)

11 BENEFITS OF ALMOND MILK DID YOU KNOW ABOUT-LIFEHACK
www.lifehack.org/articles//lifestyle/benefits-almond-mild.html (30)

TOFU-THE WORLD'S HEALTHIEST FOOD
www.whfoods.com/genpage.php?tname+foodspiceandbid=111 (31)

THE HEALTH BENEFITS OF TOFU// GOOD FOOD
www.bbcgoodfood.com/howto/guide/ingredient-focue-tofu
(32)

HORSERADISH NUTRITION FACTS AND HEALTH BENEFITS-NUTRITION
AND YOU
www.nutrition-and-you.com/horseradish.html (33)

SOY SAUCE-THE WORLD'S HEALTHEST FOODS
wwwwhfoods.com/genpage.php?thename-foodspicebid-110 (34)

11-PROVEN-BENEFITS-OF-GARLIC-AUTHORITY NUTRITION
https://authoritynutrition.com/11-proven-benefits-of-garlic/
(35)

12 HEALTH BENEFITS OF AVOCADOS
https://authoritynutriton.com/12-proven-benefits-of-benefits
(36)

THE-AMAZING-BENEFITS-OF-DRINKING-DAILY TOMATO JUICE
www.naturebacks.com/the-amazing-benefits-of-drinking-daily-tomato-juice (37)

16 HEALTH BENEFITS OF LEMONS|CARE 2 HEALTHY LIVING
www.care2.com/greenliving/16-health-benefits-of-lemons.html (38)

BENEFITS OF WHEAT GERM|ORGANIC FACTS
https://www.organicfactsnet> (39)

TURMERIC – THE WORLD'S HEALTHIEST FOODS
www.whfoods.com/genpage.php?tname-foodspice&bdid-78
(40)

PAR D' ARCO BENEFITS
www.paudarco.org/benefits.php (41)

17 BENEFITS OF CAYENNE PEPPER
www.globalhealingcenter.com/natural-health-benefits-of-cayenepepper/ (42)

CAYENNE PEPPER BENEFITS YOUR GUT, HEART, AND BEYOND – DR.
AXE
https:///draxe.com/cayenne-pepper-benefits/ (43)

OLIVE-OIL-NUTRITION-FACTS-AND-HEALTH-BENEFITS
www.nutrition-and-you.com/olive-oil.html (44)

LECITHIN – WHAT ARE THE HEALTH BENEFITS?
www.reference.com>health>medications-and-vitamins
(45)

LECITHIN – RESTORES NERVOUS CELL FUNCTION
santegrausa.com/lecithin-intensifies-metabolism-in-the-brain-cells-restores-
nerve-ce... (46)

FIGS-THE WORLD'S HEALTHIEST BENEFITS
www.whfoods.com/genpage.php?tname=foodspice&dbid=24
(47)

HEALTH BENEFITS OF DATE-OVER 7 REASONS TO EAT A DATE
FRUIT/NATURAL
naturalsociety.com/health-benefits-of-dates-7-reasons-eat-date-fruit/ (48)

5 BLACKSTRAP MOLASSES BENEFITS-HEALTHLINE
www.healthlinecom>food-and-nutrition (49)

RAISINS NUTRITION FACTS AND HEALTH BENEFITS-NUTRITION AND
YOU
www.nutrition-and-you.com/raisins.html (50)

PRUNES-HEALTH-BENEFITS-OF-PRUNES-AND-FIVE REASONS-TO-EAT-
MORE-OF-THEM
www.chatetaine.com (51)

THE IMPORTANCE OF NUTRITIONAL YEAST TO YOUR HEALTH –
MERCOLA ARTICLES
articles.mercola.com/sites/articles/archive/2016/04/04/
nutritional-yeast.aspx (52)

WHAT IS THE DIFFERENCE BETWEEN BREWER'S YEAST AND
BREWER'S YEAST?
Www.livestrog.com>Foods And Drink (53)

9 HEALTH BENEFITS OF EATING OATS AND OATMEAL
http://authoritynutrition.com/9-benefits-oats-oatmeal (54)

11 BENEFITS OF CHIA SEEDS – AUTHORITY NUTRITION
www.webmd.wcbms.com/diet/features/truth-about-chia (55)

TOP 10 QUINOA NUTRITION FACTS AND
BENEITS – DR. AXE
https://draxe.com/10.quiona-nutrition-facts-benefits/ (56)

10 FLAXSEED BENEFITS AND NUTRITION FACTS – DR. AXE
https://draxecom/10-flaxseed-benefits-nutrition-facts/ (57)

10 REASONS WHY BROWN RICE IS THE HEALTHY CHOICE –
VEGKITCHEN.COM
www.vegkitchen.com/nutrition/10-reasons-why-brown-rice-is-the-healthy-choice/
(58)

 MILLET – WORLD'S HEALTHIEST FOODS
www.whfoods.com/genpage.php?+name=53 (59)

WHAT ARE THE HEALTHIEST BENEFITS OF COUSCOUS? |
LIVESTRONG.COM
www.livestrong.com/article/440051-what-are-the-health-benefits-of-cousous./ (60)

WHAT ARE THE HEALTH BENEFITS?THE WHOLE GRAINS COUNCIL
wholegrainscouncil.org>Health Studies 101> Health Studies & Health Benefits
(61)

BLACK PEPPER – THE WORLD'S HEALTHIEST FOODS
www.whfoods.com/genpage.php?name=foodspice&dbid=74 (62)

GROUND CUMIN HEALTH BENEFITS|LIVESTRONG.COM
www.livestrong.com>Food and Drink (63)

THE SALT MYTH – HOW MUCH SODIUM SHOULD YOU EAT PER DAY?
https://authoritynutrition.com/how-much-sodium-per-day
(64)

SALT|HEALTH TOPICS|NUTRITION FACTS.ORG
nutritionFacts.org>Videos (65)

WHAT ARE THE HEALTH BENEFITS OF ONION POWDER?|HEALTHY
EATING|SF GATE
 healthyeating.sfgate.com>Nutrition>nutrition.in Food
 (66)

APPLES 101: NUTRITION FACTS AND HEALTH BENEFITS –
AUTHORITY.COM
https://authoritynutrition.com/food/apples/ (67)

CALORIES IN APPLE CIDER VINEGAR AND NUTRITION FACTS –
FatSecret
www.fatsecret.com/calories-nutrition/heinz/apple-cider- vinegar?frc (68)

HOW TO USE ACV FOR WEIGHT LOSS
www.healthyandnaturalworld.com/how-to-use
-cider-vinegar-for-weight-loss/ (69)

ORANGES 101: NUTRITION FACTS AND HEALTH BENEFITS –
AUTHORITY NUTRITION
https://authoritynutritioncom/foods/oranges (70)

ASK THE EXPERT ABOUT CANOLA OIL|THE NUTRITION SOURCE
https://www..hsph.arvard.edu>...>NutritionNews>Ask The Expert (71)

MUSHROOMS: HEALTH BENEFITS,
FACTS, RESEARCH – MEDICAL NEWS TODAY
www.medicalnewstoday.com/articles/278858.php (72)

GRAPES NUTRITION.FACTS – GRAPES NUTRITIONAL VALUE – SUN
WORLD
www.sun-world.com/grapes-nutrition (73)

7 BEST HEALTH BENEFITS OF KALE – DR. AXE
http://draxe.com/health-benefits-of-kale (74)

SPINACH – THE WORLD'S HEALTHIEST FOODS
www.whfoods.com/genpage.php?tname=foodspice&dbid-43
(75)

SPINACH 101:NUTRITION FACTS AND HEALTH BENEFITS –
AUTHORITY NUTRITION
http://authority.com/foods/spinach/ (76)

8 AMAZING HEALTH BENEFITS OF
CAULIFLOWER – MERCOLA ARTICLES – DR. MERCOLA
articles.mercola.com/sites/articles/archives/
2014/02/...cauliflower-benefits.aspx (77)

BROCCOLI 101: NUTRITION FACTS AND HEALTH BENEFITS –
AUTHORITY NUTRITION
http://authoritnutrition.com/foods/broccoli (78)

CABBAGE – THE WORLD'S HEALTHIEST FOODS
www.whfoods.com/genpage.php?tname=foodspice&bdid=19
(79)

CRUCIFEROUS VEGETABLES AND CANCER PREVENTION – NATIONAL
CANCER ...
https://www.cancer.gen/aboutcancer/causes.../risk/.../
cruciferous-vegetables-fact-sheet (80)

SULFUR -THE 4TH MAJOR NUTRIENT|NUTRIENT STEWARDSHIP
www.nutrientstewardship.com/implementation/article/
sulfur-4th-major-nutrient (81)

WATERMELON 101: NUTRITION FACTS AND HEALTH BENEFITS –
AUTHORITY NUTRITION
https://authoritynutrition.com/foods/watermelon/ (82)

CARROTS 101: NUTRITION FACTS AND HEALTH BENEFITS –
AUTHORITY NUTRITION
https://authoritynutrition.com/foods/carrots/ (83)

10 BENEFITS OF CELERY+NUTRITION FACTS AND RECEIPES – DR. AXE
https://draxe.com/benefits-of-celery (84)

ARE DILL PICKLES GOOD FOR YOU|HEALTHY EATING|SFGATE
healthyeating.afgatecom>HealthyFoodChoices (85)

20 AMAZING HEALTH BENEFITS OF TOMATOES THAT SHOULD MAKE
THEM A DAILY STAPLE IN YOUR DIET
https://healthimpactnews.com/.../20-amazing-health
benefits-of-tomatoes-that-should... (86)

ONION: THE HEALTH BENEFITS OF ONIONS
articles.mercola.com/sites/articles/archive/2016/01/04/health
benefits-onions-aspx (87)

BELL PEPPER 101: NUTRITION FACTS AND HEALTH BENEFITS
https://authoritynutrition.com/foods/bell-peppers/ (88)

POTATOES 101: NUTRITION FACTS AND HEALTH EFFECTS –
AUTHORITY NUTRITION
https://authoritynutrition.com/foods/potatoes/ (89)

13 BENEFITS OF COFFEE, BASED ON SCIENCE – AUTHORITY
NUTRITION
https://authoritynutrition.com/top-13-evidence-based-health-benefits-of-coffee/
(90)

7 PROVEN HEALTH BENEFITS OF DARK CHOCOLATE AUTHORITY
NUTRITION
https://authoritynutritioncom/7-health-benefits-dark-chocolate (91)

BLACKBERRY FACTS: 10 THINGS YOU MAY NOT KNOW ABOUT THE
FRUIT
www.huffingtonpost.ca/2013/31/blackberryfacts_n_2581622.html (92)

BLACKBERRY NUTRITION – DRISCOLL'S
https://www.driscolls.com/berries/blackberries/nutrition (93)

TANNINS|LATEST HEALTH NEWS|MEDBIZTV
www.medibiz.com/articles/health-benefits-of-plant-tannins (94)

ANTIOXIDANT|DEFINITION OF ANTIOXIDANT BY MERRIAM-WEBSTER
https://www.merriam-webster.com/dictionary/antioxidant
(95)

BENEFITS OF ANTIOXIDANTS - HOW DO ANTIOXIDANTS KEEP YOU
HEALTHY?
www.nutrex-hawaii.com/benefits-of-antioxidants (96)

WHAT ARE FREE RADICALS?
www.livescience.com>PureScience (97)

WHAT IS A FREE RADICAL? - LIVE SCIENCE
www.livescience.com>PureScience (98)

WHAT IS OXIDATIVE STRESS? - NEWS MEDICAL
www.news-medical.net/health/what-is-oxidative-stress.aspx
(99)

FACT SHEETS FOR BLACKBERRIES, BLUEBERRIES, RASPBERRIES
AND ...
berryhealth.fst.oreganstate.edu/health_healthy/fact_sheets/
(100)

RASPBERRIES – THE WORLD'S HEALTHIEST FOODS
www.whfoods.com/genpage.php?tname=foodspice&dbid=39
(101)

10 PROVEN HEALTH BENEFITS OF BLUEBERRIES – AUTHORITY
NUTRITION
http://authoritynutrition.com/10-proven-benefits-of-blueberries (102)

OLIVE 101: NUTRITION FACTS AND HEALTH BENEFITS – AUTHORITY
NUTRITION
https://authoritynutrition.com/foods/olives (103)

ACRYLAMIDE FOOD AND CANCER RISK NATIONAL CANCER
INSTITUTE
https://www.cancer.gen/about-cancerprevention/risk/.../acrylamide-fact-sheet (104)

SURPRISING FACTS ABOUT THE NUTRITIONAL VALUE OF CORN – DR.
AXE
https://draxe.com/nutritional-value-of-corn (105)

CORN 101: NUTRITION FACTS AND HEALTH BENEFITS – AUTHORITY
NUTRITION
https://authoritynutrition.com/foods/corn/ (106)

7 PROVEN BENEFITS OF QUERCERIN IS INCREDIBLE– DR. AXE
https://draxe.com/quercerin (107)

10 HEALTH BENEFITS OF PEAS|REAL FOOD FOR LIFE
www.realfoodforlife.com>nutrition (108)

ALMOND BUTTER NUTRITON INFORMATION/LIVESTRONG.COM
wwwlivestrong.com>FoodandDrink (109)

9 AMAZING BENEFITS OF ALMONDS NUTRITION – DR. AXE
https://draxe.com/almonds-nutrition/ (110)

PEANUTS – THE WORLD'S HEALTHIEST FOODS
www.whfoods.com/genpage.php?tname-foodspice&dbid=101
(111)

THE BENEFITS OF PEANUT BUTTER – PREVENTATION
www.prevention.com/food/smart.../healthy-eating-why-peanut-butter-good-you
(112)

7 BENEFITS OF WALNUTS|WALNUT NUTRITION
articles.mercola.com/sites/articles/archives/2014/06/19/7-walnuts-benefits.aspx
(113)

MACADAMIA NUT NUTRITION FACTS HEALTH BENEFITS – NUTRITION
AND YOU
www.nutrition-and-you.com/macadamia-nut.html (114)

HAZELNUTS:7 BENEFITS OF THESE HEART-HEALTHY, BRAIN,
BOOSTING NUTS.../DR. AXE
https://draxe.com/hazelnuts (115)

HEALTH BENEFITS OF BRAZIL NUTS - THE ANTI-CANCER SUPERFOOD
theshawnstevensonmodel.com/benefits-of-brazil-nuts/ (116)

FOUR BRAZIL NUTS ONCE A MONTH.../NUTRITION FACTS.ORG
nutritionfacts.org>Dr. Greger's Medical Nutrition Blog (117)

ENZYME|DEFINITION OF ENZYMATIC BY MERRIAM-WEBSTER
http://www.merriam-webster.com/dictionary/enzymatic (118)

IMPORTANCE OF ENZYMES:METABOLIC ENZYMES DIGESTIVE
ENZYMES
www.barleymagic.com/enzymes.html (119)

15 BENEFITS OF PECANS – HUDSON PECAN
www.Ilovepecan.org/nutrition-in-a-shell (120)

9 AMAZING HEALTH BENEFITS OF PUMPKIN SEEDS
articles.mercola.com/sites/article/archives/2013/09/30/
pumpkin-seed-benefits.aspx (121)

5 HEALTHY BENEFITS OF SUNFLOWER SEEDS – GLOBAL HEALING CENTER
www.globalhealingcenter.com/natural-health/health-benefits-of-sunflower-seeds/ (122)

10 PROVEN BENEFITS OF GREEN TEA – AUTHORITY NUTRITION
https://authoritynutrition.com/top-10-evidence-based-health-benefits-of-green-tea/ (123)

BENEFITS OF PEPPERMINT TEA|HEALTH GUIDE
www.newsbenefitsguide.org/Benefits-Of-Peppermint-Tea.html (124)

MINT: HEALTH BENEFITS, USES, AND RISKS – MEDICAL NEWS TODAY
www.medicalnewstoday.com/articles/275944.php (125)

CHAI TEA LATTE HEALTH BENEFITS|LIVE WELL-JILLIAN MICHAELS
livewell.jillianmichaels.com/chai-tea-latte-health-benefits-5457.html (126)

SMOOTH MOVE – TRADITIONAL MEDICINALS
www.traditionalmedicinals.com/products/smooth-more/ (127)

SAUCE, PASTA, MARINARA – ready-to-serve NUTRTIONFACTS...
nutritiondata.self.com/soups-sauces-and-gravies/1316/2 (128)

HOW LYCOPENE HELPS PROTECT AGAINST CANCER|THE PHYSCIAN ...
www.pcrm.org/health/cancer-resources/.../how-lycopene-helps-protect-against-cancer (129)

7 LYCOPENE BENEFITS THAT FIGHT DISEASE AND IMPROVE COGNITION – DR. AXE
https.//draxe.com/lycopene (130)

CALORIES IN SALSA AND NUTRIRION FACTS - FAT SECRET
https.//www.fatsecret.com/calories-nutrition/generic/salsa (131)

SALSA GIVE DIET A HEALTHY KICK – HEALTH – DIET AND NUTRITION – NUTRITION
www.nbcnews/com/id/.../...nutrition/t/salsa-grows-conbination-healthy-side-dish/ (132)

BRAGG'S APPLE CIDER VINEGAR
bragg.com/products/bragg-organic-apple-cider-vinegar.html (133)

WHAT ARE THE BENEFITS OF MOTHER OF VINEGAR?www.livestrong.com>foodand drink (134)

6 EVIDENCE – BASED HEALTH BENEFITS OF HEMP SEEDS- AUTHORTIY NUTRITION
https://authoritynutrition.com/6-health-benefits-of-hemp-seeds/ (135)

9 AMAZING HEALTH BENEFITS OF CUCUMBERS – MERCOLA ANTIOXIDANT – DR. MERCOLA
articles.mercola.com/sites/articles/archives/2014/08/.../health-benefits-cucumbers.aspx (136)

BENEFITS 101:NUTRITIONAL FACTS AND HEALTH BENEFITS – AUTHORITY NUTRITION
https://authoritynutrition.com/foods/bananas (137)

CASHEWS NUTRITION: HELPS PREVENT CANCER, DIABETES, AND MORE – DR. AXE
https://draxe.com/cashews-nutrition (138)

WHAT ARE PROBIOTICS? BENEFITS, SUPPLEMENTS, FOODS, AND MORE - WEBMD
www.webmd.com/digestive-disorders/features/what-are-probiotics (139)

RICE 101: NUTRITION AND HEALTH FACTS – HEALTHY NUTRITION
https://authoritynutrition.com/foods/rice/(140)

WHAT ARE THE BENEFITS OF SPAGHETTI?|LIVESTRONG.COM
www.livestrong.com/article/12565-what-are-the-benefits-of-spaghetti-/(141)

CALORIES IN VEGAN BREAD|NUTRITION HEALTH FACTS
https://www.caloriecount.com/vegan-bread-receipe-r545885 (142)

BRUSSEL SPROUTS – THE WORLD'S HEALTHIEST FOODS
www.whfoods.com/genpage.php?tname=foodspice&dbid=10 (143)

VEGAN | DEFINE VEGAN AT DICTIONARY.COM
www.dictionary.com/browse/vegan (144)

8 HEALTH BENEFITS OF EATING NUTS – AUTHORITY NUTRITION
https://authoritynutrition.com/8-benefits-of-nuts/ (145)

VEGANAISE|FOLLOW YOUR HEART
followyourheart.com/taq-products/veganaise (146)

Popcorn Nutrition Facts|A Healthy Low-Calorie Snack?
https://authoritynutrition.com/popcorn-nutrition-and-health/ (147)

Difference Between Purified And Distilled Water
www.endless/waters.com/distilled-or-purified-water (148)

Although this is THE END of the book, I hope it will be THE BEGINNING of health for, at least, one person who reads it.